METABOLIC DIET FOR WOMEN OVER 50

Effective 10 Days Sample Meal plan for Breakfast, Lunch, Snacks and Dinner with Delicious Recipes & Easy Exercises For Weight Loss & Healthy Lifestyle

Dr. Martins Sant

Copyright © 2023

All Rights Are Reserved

The content in this book may not be reproduced, duplicated, or transferred without the express written permission of the author or publisher. Under no circumstances will the publisher or author be held liable or legally responsible for any losses, expenditures, or damages incurred directly or indirectly as a consequence of the information included in this book.

Legal Remarks

Copyright protection applies to this publication. It is only intended for personal use. No piece of this work may be modified, distributed, sold, quoted, or paraphrased without the author's or publisher's consent.

Disclaimer Statement

Please keep in mind that the contents of this booklet are meant for educational and recreational purposes. Every effort has been made to offer accurate, up-to-date, reliable, and thorough information. There are, however, no stated or implied assurances of any kind. Readers understand that the author is providing competent counsel. The content in this book originates from several sources. Please seek the opinion of a competent professional before using any of the tactics outlined in this book. By reading this book, the reader agrees that the author will not be held accountable for any direct or indirect damages resulting from the use of the information contained therein, including, but not limited to, errors, omissions, or inaccuracies.

About The Author

Dr. Martins Sant is not just a name; he's your dedicated partner on the journey to a healthier and happier you. With over a decade of experience as a distinguished Nutritionist and Dietitian, Dr. Sant has helped countless individuals transform their lives through the power of proper nutrition.

Armed with a Master's Degree in Nutrition, Dr. Sant's expertise extends far beyond the classroom. He combines his extensive academic knowledge with a profound passion for wellness to create practical and personalized nutrition plans that bring tangible results.

He is on a mission to empower you with the knowledge and tools to make informed dietary choices that enhance your vitality, longevity, and overall well-being. Dr. Sant understands that every person is unique, and he tailors his guidance to suit your individual needs and goals.

Whether you're looking to shed those extra pounds, manage chronic health conditions, or simply adopt a balanced and nutritious lifestyle, Dr. Martins Sant is your go-to expert. His compassionate and approachable demeanor, coupled with a deep commitment to your success, make him a trusted advisor you can rely on.

Join Dr. Sant on a journey to unlock the secrets of nourishing your body and achieving the best version of yourself. With his guidance, you'll discover that optimal health is within your reach, and a fulfilling, nutritious life is just a choice away.

TABLE OF CONTENTS

INTRODUCTION

Welcome to the incredible journey of using the Metabolic Diet, which is designed especially for women over 50, to restore your health and vitality. This book is your reliable guide to a healthier, livelier, and more satisfying life—it's more than just a compilation of recipes and meal ideas.

As we age, metabolism—the subtle engine that powers your body—often takes center stage. But do not be alarmed; this is not a story of impending doom. Rather, it's a narrative of empowerment, understanding, and metamorphosis.

Imagine your metabolism as a finely tuned orchestra, with each part contributing significantly to the overall symphony of life. Even though this orchestra is going into its golden years, it can still create lovely harmonies under the direction of a skilled director like you.

You will delve into the science of metabolism in these pages, learning about the complexities of your body's energy metabolism and why it varies with age. You'll get an appreciation for the grace of balance as we examine the complex interactions that exist between hormones, foods, and exercise.

But theory is not the only topic in this book. It's a useful manual for controlling your metabolic fate. There, you'll get practical guidance on creating a customized metabolic diet, along with mouthwatering recipes and meal planning. This is about embracing healthy, fulfilling, and nutritious foods—not about deprivation or irrational expectations.

You'll learn the value of exercise as a means of igniting your metabolic fire as well as a tool for weight loss. We'll lead you through routines and exercises designed specifically to meet the needs and goals of ladies over fifty.

You'll discover the secrets of hormones, which are frequently the unseen masterminds behind metabolic shifts, and how to cooperate with them instead of fighting them. Menopause, once a scary change in life, can now be welcomed as a life-changing event.

Your progress may slow due to obstacles and plateaus, but we'll provide you with the means to get beyond them and continue to have an enjoyable and fulfilling journey.

This book is a compass for a lifetime of vigorous living, not just a collection of quick fixes. We'll walk you through the steps to not only achieve metabolic health but also keep it there, so you can enjoy the results of years of hard work and devotion.

Together, we set out on a path to create a life of restored energy by balancing science, diet, exercise, and self-care. Your metabolic vitality holds the key to opening doors to an abundance of energy, glowing health, and self-assurance to enjoy your prime years.

Turn the page, spark your curiosity, and let's embark on this illuminating journey towards a more vivid and powerful you, dear reader. You are invited to join the waiting symphony of health and well-being that is the Metabolic Diet for Women Over 50.

CHAPTER ONE

THE SCIENCE OF METABOLISM

Exploring the basics of metabolism

Let's examine the fundamentals of metabolism, which is the process that powers your body and supplies the energy required for all bodily functions, including breathing and marathon running. Your cells go through a complicated and intriguing series of chemical events called metabolism.

What Is Metabolism?

All of the chemical processes your body goes through to stay alive are referred to as metabolism. The two primary categories of these reactions are anabolism and catabolism.

1. Decomposition: In this stage of metabolism, complex molecules are broken down into simpler ones. One example of a catabolic process is the breakdown of food in your stomach and intestines. It releases bioavailable energy and tiny chemicals into your body.

2. Abolition: On the other hand, anabolism is a group of metabolic activities that transform simpler molecules into complex ones. It is involved, for example, in the synthesis of proteins, DNA, and other macromolecules needed for development and repair.

Production of Energy:

The generation of energy is among metabolism's most important functions. Your diet provides your body with energy, mostly in the form of lipids and glucose. This is how the procedure operates:

Protection: Glycolysis is the process by which glucose is broken down into pyruvate and releases a small quantity of energy in the cytoplasm of your cells.

Citric Acid Cycle:

Krebs Cycle: More energy is produced when pyruvate enters the mitochondria, the cell's power plant, and is further broken down into carbon dioxide.

The Chain of Electron Transport: The mitochondria produce a substantial quantity of energy in the form of adenosine triphosphate (ATP), the body's principal energy currency, by moving electrons from glucose and lipids via a chain of proteins.

Metabolism-Related Factors:

A number of things affect your metabolic rate, or the speed at which your body burns calories:

Size: As we age, our metabolism naturally slows down. Because of this, it's critical to modify your diet and way of life as you age.

Physical Make-Up: Calorie-burning muscle burns more than fat. Therefore, people with more muscular mass tend to have higher metabolic rates.

Hereditary: Your metabolic rate is influenced by your genetic composition. Certain individuals may inherently possess a quicker or slower metabolism.

Sensations: Insulin and thyroid hormones, for example, have a big influence on metabolism. The total metabolic rate is regulated by thyroid hormones, while blood sugar levels are regulated by insulin.

Nutrition and Exercise: Your metabolic rate is directly influenced by what you consume and how active you are. Maintaining or raising your metabolism can be facilitated by a healthy diet and consistent exercise.

How metabolism changes with age

Understanding these changes is essential to preserving your best health and successfully managing your weight. As we age, our metabolisms naturally alter.

1. Younger Years:

- **Basal Metabolic Rate (BMR):** Your BMR is often higher while you're younger. BMR is the rate at which your body uses energy to sustain essential bodily processes, such as breathing and temperature regulation, while at rest.

- **Influence of Aging:** Your BMR normally drops with age. Loss of muscle mass, which is more metabolically active and consumes calories than fat, is the main cause of this. The aging process naturally involves the loss of muscular tissue, which slows down metabolism over time.

2. Hormonal Shifts:

- **Earlier Ages:** The regulation of metabolism is significantly influenced by hormones. Hormone balance is often better in youth, which supports a healthy metabolic rate.

- **Influence of Aging:** Hormone production varies with age, particularly in women going through menopause and in males going through andropause. Changes in hormones can cause an increase in body weight and a decrease in muscle mass. A reduction in estrogen in women may have an impact on fat distribution, with the abdomen storing more fat.

3. Exercise:

- **Younger Years:** Younger people typically have higher levels of physical activity, which might increase their metabolism. Frequent exercise promotes a faster metabolism and aids in the maintenance of muscular mass.

- **Influence of Aging:** People frequently become less active as they get older for a variety of reasons, such as changes in their jobs, obligations to their families, and physical limits. Decreased physical activity might worsen metabolic slowdown and cause a loss of muscle mass.

4. Nutrition and Digestion:

- **Early Years:** The body is frequently more adept at breaking down and absorbing nutrients from meals while it is young. This aids in the metabolism of energy.

- **Influence of Aging:** As we age, our digestive efficiency may decline, and our body's ability to absorb nutrients may also diminish. This may result in dietary deficits that affect metabolism and general health.

5. Lifestyle Factors:

- **youthful Years:** A lot of people in their youthful years lead more adaptable and active lives.
- **Influence of Aging:** People may modify their lifestyles as they get older, which can lower their metabolism. Retirement, a decrease in physical activity, and adjustments to daily schedules are a few examples of these changes.

Factors influencing metabolic rate

Numerous factors affect metabolic rate, which is the pace at which your body burns calories to create energy. You may manage your weight and general health by making educated decisions regarding your diet, exercise routine, and lifestyle by being aware of these issues.

1. Year:

Significance: As people age, their metabolic rate often drops. Changes in hormone levels and a decline in muscle mass are the main causes of this. In general, younger people have a greater metabolic rate than elderly people.

2. Mass of Muscle:

Impact: Compared to fat tissue, muscle tissue has a higher resting metabolic rate and consumes more calories. Your basal metabolic rate may rise if you have greater muscle mass (BMR). As a result, people who have a larger percentage of muscle typically have faster metabolisms.

3. Sex:

Importance: Because they typically have less body fat and more muscular mass than women, men often have higher BMRs than women. Variations in hormones also come into play.

4.Impact:

Hormones: Insulin and thyroid hormones are two examples of hormones that are important in controlling metabolism. The thyroid gland produces thyroid hormones, which have an impact on the total metabolic rate. Insulin can impact how your body uses and stores energy, in addition to helping to control blood sugar levels.

5. Nutrition and Diet:

Result: Your metabolism is directly impacted by the stuff you eat. It's crucial to consume enough calories to meet your energy requirements. A low-calorie intake may cause the metabolism to slow down in order to preserve energy. The energy used for food digestion, absorption, and storage is known as the thermic effect of food (TEF). Diets high in protein have greater TEFs, which can momentarily speed up metabolism.

6. Activities Physically:

Results: Engaging in physical activity, encompassing both strenuous and non-strenuous activities (such as standing and fidgeting), can dramatically boost metabolism and energy expenditure. Frequent exercise helps preserve muscle mass and increase BMR.

7. Hereditary:

Effect: Your metabolic rate can be somewhat influenced by your genetic composition. Because of their DNA, some people are born with a faster or slower metabolism.

8. Temperature and Environment:

Impact: Extreme temperature swings might cause your body to temporarily increase metabolism as it works harder to maintain a constant core temperature. On the other hand, prolonged exposure to very high or low temperatures can alter your metabolic rate.

9. Relaxation and Sleep:

Result: Hormonal balance can be upset by stress and sleep deprivation, which can then impact metabolism. Cortisol, which is released when a person experiences ongoing stress, may have an impact on how the body stores and uses energy.

10. Medications and Health Issues:

Result: A number of illnesses can impact metabolism, including thyroid issues and PCOS (polycystic ovarian syndrome). Drugs may also affect metabolic rate, such as Your BMR is influenced by the proportion of fat to muscle in your body. Your body composition might alter, and this can also affect your metabolic rate.

The role of hormones in metabolism

Hormones play a crucial role in regulating metabolism, influencing how your body processes and utilizes energy. These chemical messengers are produced by various glands in your body and help control many metabolic processes.

1. Thyroid Hormones (T3 and T4):

Role: The thyroid gland produces these hormones, which are essential for regulating the overall metabolic rate. They influence how your cells use energy and can affect heart rate, body temperature, and the rate at which your body burns calories.

2. Insulin:

Role: Produced by the pancreas, insulin plays a central role in regulating blood sugar levels. It enables cells to take in glucose from the bloodstream, which is used for energy or stored as glycogen in the liver and muscles. When insulin levels are well regulated, it helps control hunger and the storage of excess calories as fat.

3. Glucagon:

Role: Also produced by the pancreas, glucagon has the opposite effect of insulin. It promotes the release of stored glucose from the liver, raising blood sugar levels when they're too low. This hormone helps balance blood sugar and maintain energy levels.

4. Leptin:

Role: Leptin is produced by fat cells and plays a key role in regulating appetite and body weight. It signals to the brain when you have enough energy stored (in the form of body fat) and can help control food intake and energy expenditure.

5. Ghrelin:

Role: Ghrelin is produced by the stomach and stimulates hunger. Its levels rise before meals and fall after eating, influencing meal initiation. It can also affect fat storage and metabolism.

6. Cortisol:

Role: Produced by the adrenal glands, cortisol is known as the "stress hormone." It helps the body deal with stress by increasing blood sugar levels and promoting the breakdown of fat and protein for energy. Prolonged stress and elevated cortisol levels can have negative effects on metabolism.

7. Epinephrine (adrenaline) and norepinephrine:

Role: Produced by the adrenal glands, these hormones are released during the "fight or flight" response. They increase heart rate, elevate blood pressure, and stimulate the breakdown of glycogen into glucose to provide a rapid source of energy.

8. Estrogen and progesterone:

Role: These female sex hormones affect fat storage and distribution. Changes in estrogen levels, particularly during menopause, can influence how fat is stored in the body. Estrogen also has a role in maintaining bone health and muscle mass, which indirectly affect metabolism.

9. Testosterone:

Role: While often associated with men, testosterone is present in both men and women, albeit in different quantities. It promotes muscle growth and helps maintain lean body mass, influencing metabolism and energy expenditure.

10. Adiponectin and Resistin:

Role: These hormones are secreted by fat tissue (adipose cells) and are involved in regulating glucose metabolism and insulin sensitivity. Adiponectin has anti-inflammatory and insulin-sensitizing effects, while resistance may contribute to insulin resistance.

CHAPTER TWO

ASSESSING YOUR METABOLIC HEALTH

Self-assessment tools and tests for metabolic health

Tests and self-assessment instruments can offer insightful information about your metabolic health. You may make more educated judgments about your nutrition, exercise routine, and lifestyle by keeping an eye on your metabolic health.

Summary: A straightforward formula called BMI compares your weight to your height. It can give you an approximate idea of whether you are underweight, normal weight, overweight, or obese, even if it doesn't evaluate metabolic health directly.

How to Apply: Numerous online calculators are available to help you calculate your BMI, depending on your height and weight. Remember that body mass index (BMI) has its limits and might not take body composition changes into consideration.

2. Hip-to-Hip Ratio (WHR):

Explanation: WHR evaluates how fat is distributed across your body. It is a more accurate measure of visceral fat, or fat adipose tissue around organs, which is linked to metabolic health.

How to Apply: Take a measurement at the narrowest spot on your waist and the widest point on your hips. Next, divide the width of your hips by the length of your waist. For women, a WHR of 0.85 or below is typically regarded as healthy.

3. Blood Pressure Monitoring:

Description: High blood pressure raises the risk of a number of metabolic diseases, such as diabetes and heart disease. Frequent observation can assist in spotting possible problems.

How to Apply: To check your blood pressure, use a home blood pressure monitor or go to the doctor. Typically, normal blood pressure is 120/80 mm Hg.

4. Blood Glucose Testing:

Description: Checking your blood glucose levels is important for metabolic health since it can reveal how well your body metabolizes carbs and regulates blood sugar.

How to Apply: In the morning, you can check your fasting blood sugar with a glucometer. Generally speaking, fasting blood sugar is less than 100 mg/dL.

Tests for hemoglobin A1c offer a longer-term perspective on blood sugar regulation; levels less than 5.7% are generally regarded as healthy.

5. Cholesterol Panel Lipid Profile: The purpose of this test is to determine your blood's triglyceride and cholesterol levels, which can give you an idea of how likely you are to develop heart disease.

How to Apply:

Triglycerides, HDL (high-density lipoprotein) cholesterol, LDL (low-density lipoprotein) cholesterol, and total cholesterol are all measured as part of a lipid profile. Individual health considerations determine the optimal values for each component.

6. Metabolic Syndrome Assessment:

Description: A group of risk factors known as metabolic syndrome raises the possibility of heart disease, diabetes, and stroke. If you have many risk factors for metabolic syndrome, such as a large waist circumference, high blood pressure, high triglycerides, low HDL cholesterol, and high fasting blood sugar, you can self-evaluate for the condition.

How to Use: Speak with your doctor about your risk factors and have the necessary testing done.

7. Caloric Needs Assessment

Description: You can adjust your diet to support metabolic health and maintain a healthy weight by being aware of your daily caloric needs.

How to Apply: Your daily calorie requirements can be estimated using applications and online calculators, depending on your goals, age, gender, weight, and degree of activity.

8. Food and Activity Journals

Description: Maintaining a record of your food intake and physical activity can help you pinpoint areas for improvement by offering insights into your eating and exercise habits.

How to Apply: For a few days or weeks, keep a journal of your food intake, portion sizes, and physical activity. Examine your journal to spot patterns and make any necessary corrections.

Identifying risk factors and potential issues

Identifying risk factors and potential issues related to metabolic health is a proactive step in preventing and managing metabolic conditions. By recognizing these factors early, you can take appropriate measures to reduce your risk and promote better metabolic health. Here are some key risk factors and potential issues to consider:

1. Age:

- **Risk Factor:** Aging is a natural risk factor for metabolic changes, such as a decrease in muscle mass and a slower metabolism.
- **Potential Issue:** As you get older, it's essential to be aware of these changes and make adjustments to your diet and exercise routines to support metabolic health.

2. Excess Body Weight:

- **Risk Factor:** Being overweight or obese is a significant risk factor for metabolic conditions, including insulin resistance, type 2 diabetes, and cardiovascular disease.
- **Potential Issue:** Excess body weight can contribute to inflammation and hormonal imbalances that affect metabolic health. Addressing weight management is crucial for reducing these risks.

3. Unhealthy Diet:

- **Risk Factor:** A diet high in processed foods, added sugars, saturated fats, and nutrients can lead to metabolic issues, including insulin resistance and obesity.

- **Potential Issue:** Poor dietary choices can increase inflammation and the risk of metabolic syndrome. Evaluating and improving your dietary habits can make a significant difference.

4. Sedentary Lifestyle:

- **Risk Factor:** Lack of physical activity and prolonged periods of sitting can contribute to metabolic problems, including weight gain and insulin resistance.

- **Potential Issue:** Regular exercise can boost metabolism, improve insulin sensitivity, and support overall metabolic health. Make an effort to incorporate physical activity into your daily routine.

5. Genetics:

- **Risk Factor:** A family history of metabolic conditions like diabetes or obesity can increase your risk of developing similar issues.

- **Potential Issue:** Understanding your genetic predispositions can help you be proactive in managing your metabolic health and seeking early intervention if necessary.

6. Hormonal Changes:

- **Risk Factor:** Hormonal fluctuations, such as those occurring during menopause in women or andropause in men, can impact metabolic health.
- **Potential Issue:** Recognizing these changes and discussing them with a healthcare provider can lead to tailored strategies for managing metabolic health.

7. Stress:

- **Risk Factor:** Chronic stress can lead to the release of cortisol, which may influence how your body stores and uses energy.
- **Potential Issue:** Managing stress through relaxation techniques, exercise, and lifestyle changes can positively impact metabolic health.

8. Sleep Problems:

Risk Factor: Inadequate or poor-quality sleep can disrupt hormones that regulate appetite and metabolism.

Potential Issue: Prioritizing good sleep hygiene and seeking treatment for sleep disorders can help maintain metabolic health.

9. Existing Health Conditions:

- **Risk Factor:** Certain medical conditions, such as polycystic ovary syndrome (PCOS), thyroid disorders, and metabolic syndrome, are associated with metabolic issues.

- **Potential Issue:** Managing these conditions with the guidance of a healthcare provider is crucial for maintaining metabolic health.

10. Medications:

- **Risk Factor:** Some medications, including certain antidepressants and steroids, can affect metabolic rate and contribute to weight gain.

- **Potential Issue:** Discuss any concerns about medication-related metabolic changes with your healthcare provider.

Working with healthcare professionals to evaluate your metabolic health

A smart and proactive way to comprehend and manage your health is to collaborate with healthcare professionals to assess your metabolic health.

1. Select the Appropriate Medical Team:

Primary Care Physician: Speak with your primary care provider first. They can arrange for your medical care and act as your initial point of contact.

Experts: You might need to speak with experts like exercise physiologists, dietitians, or nutritionists, as well as endocrinologists, depending on your particular needs.

2. Plan Observational Examinations:

Medical Examinations: Don't forget to arrange routine examinations with your primary care provider. Talk to your doctor about any potential risk factors and any concerns regarding your metabolic health throughout these sessions.

3. Health and Family Background:

Give Detailed Information: Please provide your medical history, taking into account any current ailments, prescription drugs, and any family history of metabolic diseases like diabetes or obesity.

4. Risk Factor Assessment:

Physical Examination: To evaluate your general health, your healthcare professional will perform a physical examination. This could entail taking your blood pressure, height, and weight.

Heart Exams: Blood tests may be performed on you to assess a number of factors, including thyroid function, lipid profile, and fasting blood sugar. The results of these tests can provide important insights into your metabolic health.

5. Lifestyle Evaluation:

Nutrition and Exercise: Talk to your healthcare professional about your lifestyle choices, exercise regimen, and food habits. Tell the truth about your food habits and amount of physical activity.

Relaxation and Stress: Bring up any sleep issues or ongoing stress you may be dealing with, as they might affect metabolic health.

6. Personalized Assessment:

Evaluation: Your healthcare practitioner will conduct a personalized review based on your medical history and test results to determine any metabolic problems or risk factors unique to your circumstances.

7. Metabolic Conditions Screening:

Diabetes Screening: Your healthcare practitioner may conduct further tests, such as an oral glucose tolerance test or a hemoglobin A1c test, if you have risk factors for diabetes.

Checking for Additional Conditions: You might undergo screening for diseases like polycystic ovarian syndrome (PCOS) or thyroid abnormalities based on your medical history and risk factors.

8. Cooperative Objective-Setting:

Talk about the objectives: Set attainable health goals in collaboration with your healthcare professional. These could be controlling your weight, making dietary changes, getting more exercise, or taking care of any health issues you already have.

9. Recommendations for Treatment and Lifestyle:

Medication, if Required: In the event that metabolic

disorders are identified, your physician can suggest taking medication to treat them.

Changes to Lifestyle: It is likely that you may be given advice on dietary and lifestyle modifications that will enhance metabolic health. This can include suggestions for stress reduction, exercise, and a balanced diet.

10. Monitoring and Follow-up:

Regular Inspections: As advised by your healthcare professional, establish follow-up appointments so that you can assess your progress and modify your treatment plan as needed.

Open Interface: Maintain open channels of contact with your medical staff. You should not be afraid to ask for help and support if you encounter any changes or difficulties.

CHAPTER THREE

TAILORING YOUR DIET FOR METABOLIC HEALTH

Understanding macronutrients and micronutrients

Understanding macronutrients and micronutrients is essential for making informed dietary choices to support your overall health and well-being. These nutrients are the building blocks of your diet, and they play specific roles in your body's functions.

Macronutrients:

Macronutrients are nutrients that your body requires in larger quantities for energy, growth, and everyday functions. There are three primary macronutrients:

1. Carbohydrates:

Function: Carbohydrates are the body's primary source of energy. They are broken down into glucose, which is used to fuel various bodily processes.

Sources: Carbohydrates are found in foods like grains, bread, pasta, rice, fruits, vegetables, and legumes.

2. Proteins:

Function: Proteins are essential for the growth, repair, and maintenance of body tissues. They are also involved in enzyme production, immune function, and hormone production.

Sources: Protein-rich foods include lean meats, poultry, fish, eggs, dairy products, legumes, nuts, and seeds.

3. Fats:

Function: Fats provide a concentrated source of energy and play a crucial role in protecting organs, insulating the body, and absorbing fat-soluble vitamins (micronutrients).

Sources: Healthy sources of fats include avocados, nuts, seeds, olive oil, fatty fish, and dairy products. Unsaturated fats are preferred over saturated and trans fats.

Micronutrients:

Micronutrients are nutrients that your body needs in smaller quantities to maintain health and perform various functions. There are two primary categories of micronutrients:

1. Vitamins:

Function: Vitamins are organic compounds that serve as coenzymes in various metabolic reactions. They play vital roles in immune function, energy production, and overall health.

Sources: Vitamins are found in a wide range of foods, including fruits, vegetables, whole grains, dairy products, and lean protein sources. Each vitamin has unique food sources.

Examples of Common Vitamins:

- Vitamin A is important for vision, immune function, and skin health.
- Vitamin C is an antioxidant that supports immune health and skin integrity.
- Vitamin D is essential for calcium absorption and bone health.
- Vitamin E is an antioxidant that helps protect cells from damage.
- Vitamin K is necessary for blood clotting and bone health.
- B vitamins (e.g., B1, B2, B3, B6, and B12) are involved in energy metabolism, nerve function, and red blood cell production.

2. Minerals:

Function: Minerals are inorganic elements that play critical roles in various physiological processes, including bone health, fluid balance, nerve function, and oxygen transport.

Sources: Minerals are found in a variety of foods, with some being particularly abundant in specific food groups. Examples include calcium in dairy products, iron in red meat, and potassium in fruits and vegetables.

Examples of Common Minerals:

- Calcium is crucial for bone health, muscle function, and blood clotting.
- Iron is essential for oxygen transport in red blood cells.
- Potassium helps regulate blood pressure and muscle contractions.
- Magnesium supports muscle and nerve function, as well as bone health.
- Zinc is important for immune function and wound healing.
- Selenium acts as an antioxidant and is vital for thyroid function.

Developing a personalized metabolic diet plan

Creating a customized metabolic diet plan entails adjusting you're eating patterns to meet your unique metabolic requirements and objectives. This program can help you control your weight, speed up your metabolism, and improve your general health.

1. Speak with a Registered Dietitian or Healthcare Provider: Seek advice from a certified dietician or healthcare physician before making any major dietary changes. They are able to evaluate the state of your health, metabolic health, and nutritional requirements.

2. Set Specific Objectives: Establish your main dietary objectives. Are you trying to manage a certain illness like diabetes, enhance metabolic health, maintain a healthy weight, or reduce weight? Your food selections will be guided by your clearly defined goals.

3. Calculate Your Caloric Needs: Determine how many calories you need each day based on your age, gender, degree of exercise, and objectives. For a more precise estimate, you can speak with a dietician or use internet calculators.

4. Balance Macronutrients: Modify the proportions of your macronutrients (fats, proteins, and carbohydrates) to suit your needs and metabolic requirements. For instance, think about eating a balanced diet that includes enough proteins, carbs, and healthy fats if your goal is to keep your blood sugar levels steady.

5. Make Whole Foods a Priority: Make whole, unprocessed foods the foundation of your diet. Make sure your diet is rich in whole grains, fruits, veggies, lean meats, and healthy fats. Whole foods are high in fiber and other important nutrients that might help maintain a healthy metabolism.

6. Select high-quality carbs: Choose complex carbs found in vegetables, whole grains, and legumes. They help control blood sugar levels and offer a consistent supply of energy.

7. Incorporate Lean Proteins: Include sources of lean protein such as fish, chicken, beans, and tofu. Both appetite control and muscle maintenance are aided by protein.

8. Select Healthy Fats: Opt for unsaturated fats, which may be found in foods such as olive oil, avocados, almonds, and seeds. These fats promote general health and heart wellness.

9. Manage Portion Dimensions: Pay attention to portion proportions to prevent overindulging. To control calorie consumption, pay attention to indications of hunger and fullness, and practice portion management.

10. Remain Hydrated: The metabolism depends on staying properly hydrated. Water is a great beverage to have throughout the day to aid with digestion and general wellness.

11. Think About Meal Timing: Eating consistent, well-balanced meals and snacks throughout the day will support steady blood sugar and energy levels. A prolonged fast might slow down metabolism, so avoid going too long without eating.

12. Keep an eye on your blood sugar levels: If blood sugar regulation worries you, you might want to try routinely monitoring your blood glucose levels, particularly after meals. This can assist in spotting any trends and directing dietary changes.

13. Fiber-Rich Foods: Make sure your diet includes foods high in fiber, such as whole grains, legumes, fruits, and vegetables. Fiber supports healthy digestion, steady blood sugar levels, and fullness.

14. Individualize Nutrient Needs: Take into account any specific nutritional requirements you might have. For instance, your dietitian might offer advice on how to meet your needs if you are deficient in vitamins or minerals.

15. Take into account medical issues: Make sure to modify your diet plan in accordance with any special dietary needs or medical issues you may have, such as celiac disease, lactose intolerance, or food allergies.

16. Regular Exercise: Make physical activity a regular part of your day. Your metabolism can be accelerated, and your weight management objectives can be supported with exercise.

17. Regular Reevaluation: Review your progress on a regular basis and modify your nutrition plan as necessary. Adaptability is key because your metabolic needs can change over time.

Balancing calories and nutrients to support a healthy metabolism

Maintaining a healthy metabolism and general wellbeing depends on maintaining a balance between calories and nutrients. A balanced diet gives your body the energy it needs to perform at its best and supplies vital nutrients for different metabolic functions.

1. Calculate Your Daily Calorie Needs: Determine your daily calorie needs by factoring in things like age, gender, degree of exercise, and objectives. You can get help with this by using online calculators or by speaking with a trained dietician.

2. Make Whole, Nutrient-Dense Foods a Priority: Make whole, minimally processed foods high in vital nutrients your first choice. Fruits, vegetables, whole grains, lean meats, nuts, seeds, and healthy fats are some of these.

3. Balance Macronutrients: Align the distribution of macronutrients (fats, proteins, and carbohydrates):

Carbs: Make whole grains, legumes, and vegetables—which are high in complex carbohydrates—your main source of energy. Eat fewer processed and sugary foods.

Semites: Incorporate lean proteins (fish, chicken, beans, and tofu) into your diet to help with satiety and muscle maintenance.

Size: Opt for unsaturated fats (found in almonds, avocados, and olive oil) rather than trans and saturated fats. Long-lasting energy and general health are supported by fats.

4. Portion Control: Be mindful of portion proportions to control calorie intake and prevent overindulging. Visual signals and measurements can be useful.

5. Regular Meals and Snacks: A constant blood sugar level can be maintained by eating regular, balanced meals and snacks. Avoid excessive hunger, however, as this might slow down the metabolism.

6. Hydration: Drink water all day long to stay well hydrated. Drinking enough water is crucial for a healthy metabolism and general wellbeing.

7. Include Fiber: Include foods high in fiber, such as whole grains, legumes, fruits, and vegetables. In addition to keeping your stomach feeling full, fiber also helps to keep blood sugar levels stable.

8. Manage Sugar Additives: Reduce the amount of added sugars in your diet because eating too much of it might cause energy surges and crashes. To find hidden sugars in packaged goods, read food labels.

9. Minerals and Vitamins: Eat a wide variety of meals to make sure your diet contains a variety of vitamins and minerals. Particularly, fruits and vegetables offer a variety of vitamins.

10. Lean Proteins: Select sources of lean protein to help maintain your general health and muscle mass. Foods high in protein also have a stronger thermic effect, which means they can marginally increase metabolism while being digested.

11. Regular Physical Activity: Make exercise a regular part of your schedule. Engaging in physical activity can increase your metabolism by maintaining and growing lean muscle.

12. Equilibrium Caloric Consumption and Intake: It's crucial to strike a balance between the calories you take in and the calories you burn from daily activities and physical exercise in order to maintain a healthy weight.

13. Mindful Eating: Pay attention to your body's signals of hunger and fullness while you eat mindfully. Steer clear of stress- or emotion-related eating since it can result in overindulgence.

14. Metabolic Health Monitoring: Consult with medical specialists to monitor and treat any specific metabolic issues or medical illnesses through dietary and lifestyle modifications.

15. Regular Reevaluation: Review your diet plan on a regular basis to make sure it helps your metabolic health and is in line with your objectives. Based on your development, modify your diet as necessary.

45

CHAPTER FOUR

THE METABOLIC DIET PLAN

Detailed guidelines for the Metabolic Diet

The goals of a metabolic diet are to maintain a healthy metabolism, control weight, and enhance general wellbeing.

1. Speak with a Medical Professional: Speak with a medical professional or a licensed dietitian before beginning any diet plan. They can evaluate your current state of health and assist in customizing your diet to meet your unique requirements.

2. Set clear goals: Establish your dietary objectives, such as controlling your weight, enhancing your metabolic health, or managing a certain medical condition.

3. Balanced Macronutrients: Align the distribution of macronutrients:

- **Carbohydrates:** To support blood sugar regulation and offer consistent energy, choose complex carbohydrates from whole grains, legumes, and vegetables.

- **Proteins:** To assist appetite control and muscle maintenance, include lean protein sources such as fish, chicken, beans, tofu, and low-fat dairy.
- **Size:** Choose unsaturated fats from foods such as olive oil, avocados, almonds, and seeds. Cut back on trans and saturated fats.

4. Portion Control: Monitor your calorie consumption by keeping an eye on portion sizes. Using visual signals or measuring meals can be beneficial.

5. Regular Meals and Snacks: Consume well-balanced meals and snacks on a regular basis to stave off severe hunger and keep blood sugar levels steady.

6. Hydration: Drink water all day long to stay well hydrated. Maintaining adequate hydration promotes a healthy metabolism and general wellbeing.

7. Fiber-Rich Foods: Include foods high in fiber, such as whole grains, legumes, fruits, and vegetables. Fiber supports healthy digestion, stable blood sugar levels, and fullness.

8. Control Added Sugars: Read food labels, stay away from sugar-filled drinks, and cut back on processed snacks to reduce added sugar intake.

9. Whole Foods: Give less processed, whole foods precedence over highly processed ones. Nutrient-dense whole foods are vital for a healthy metabolism.

10. Lean Proteins: Select sources of lean protein to help maintain your general health and muscle mass. Foods high in protein also have a stronger thermic effect, which means they can marginally increase metabolism while being digested.

11. Regular Physical Activity: Make exercise a regular part of your schedule. Engaging in physical activity can increase your metabolism by maintaining and growing lean muscle.

12. Equilibrium Caloric Consumption and Intake: You must balance the calories you eat with the calories you burn from everyday activities and physical exercise in order to maintain a healthy weight.

13. Mindful Eating: Pay attention to your body's signals of hunger and fullness while you eat mindfully. Steer clear of stress- or emotion-related eating.

14. Stress Management: Reduce stress by practicing mindfulness, working out, and making lifestyle adjustments. Hormones and metabolism can be impacted by prolonged stress.

15. Sleep: Make maintaining proper sleep hygiene a priority and strive for 7-9 hours of restful sleep every night. Hormones that control metabolism and hunger could be upset by getting too little sleep.

16. Individualized nutritional needs: Take into account your unique nutritional requirements depending on your age, gender, and any particular health issues you may be experiencing.

17. Medication Management: If you have any medical issues that call for medication, make sure the advice from your healthcare practitioner fits into your diet.

18. Metabolic Health Monitoring: Consult a healthcare provider if you have any specific metabolic issues or medical illnesses so that you can monitor and treat them with dietary and lifestyle modifications.

19. Regular Reevaluation: Review your diet plan on a regular basis to make sure it helps your metabolic health and is in line with your objectives. Based on your development, modify your diet as necessary.

Sample meal plans and recipes

Here are 10 sample meal plans along with recipes for a variety of dietary preferences. These plans are designed to support a healthy metabolism and overall well-being.

Sample Meal Plan 1: Balanced Diet

Breakfast:

- Scrambled Eggs with Spinach and Tomatoes
- Whole-grain toast
- Fresh Fruit Salad

Lunch:

- Grilled Chicken Salad with Mixed Greens, Cherry Tomatoes, and Balsamic Vinaigrette
- Quinoa

Snack:

- Greek Yogurt with Berries and Honey

Dinner:

- Baked Salmon with Lemon and Dill
- Steamed Broccoli
- Brown rice

Sample Meal Plan 2: Vegetarian

Breakfast:

- Veggie Omelette with Bell Peppers, Onions, and Spinach
- Whole Wheat Toast

Lunch:

- Chickpea and Vegetable Stir-Fry with Tofu
- Brown rice

Snack:

- Hummus with Carrot Sticks

Dinner:

- Roasted Portobello Mushrooms with Quinoa and Pesto
- Mixed Green Salad

Sample Meal Plan 3: Low-Carb

Breakfast:

- Greek Yogurt with Berries and Chia Seeds

Lunch:

- Grilled Chicken Breast with Asparagus and Lemon
- Cauliflower Mash

Snack:

- Almonds and walnuts

Dinner:

- Baked Cod with Garlic Butter
- Steamed green beans

Sample Meal Plan 4: Vegan

Breakfast:

- Overnight Oats with Almond Milk, Chia Seeds, and Fresh Fruit

Lunch:

- Lentil and vegetable stew
- Whole-grain bread

Snack:

- Sliced cucumber with hummus

Dinner:

- Chickpea Curry with Brown Rice

Sample Meal Plan 5: Mediterranean

Breakfast:

- Greek Yogurt Parfait with Honey and Walnuts

Lunch:

- Mediterranean Salad with Romaine Lettuce, Kalamata Olives, Feta Cheese, and Tzatziki Dressing

Grilled chicken

Snack:

- Sliced Red Bell Pepper with Hummus

Dinner:

- Grilled Shrimp with Lemon and Herbs
- Quinoa Pilaf with Roasted Vegetables

Sample Meal Plan 6: Gluten-Free

Breakfast:

- Scrambled Eggs with Sautéed Spinach
- Quinoa Breakfast Bowl with Berries

Lunch:

- Grilled Turkey and Avocado Lettuce Wraps

Snack:

- Mixed Nuts

Dinner:

- Baked Salmon with Dijon and Honey Glaze

- Steamed asparagus
- Wild Rice

Sample Meal Plan 7: Paleo

Breakfast:

- Sweet Potato and Bacon Breakfast Hash

Lunch:

- Grilled Chicken and Vegetable Skewers

Snack:

- Sliced apples with almond butter

Dinner:

- Baked Cod with Lemon and Garlic
- Roasted Brussels sprouts

Sample Meal Plan 8: High-Protein

Breakfast:

- Protein Pancakes with Greek Yogurt and Berries

Lunch:

- Turkey and Avocado Salad with a Balsamic Vinaigrette
- Quinoa

Snack:

- Cottage Cheese with Pineapple

Dinner:

- Grilled Steak with Chimichurri Sauce
- Steamed Broccoli
- Mashed sweet potatoes

Sample Meal Plan 9: Quick and Easy

Breakfast:

- Peanut Butter and Banana Smoothie

Lunch:

- Turkey and Avocado Wrap

Snack:

- Baby Carrots with Hummus

Dinner:

- Teriyaki Chicken Stir-Fry with Vegetables

Sample Meal Plan 10: Budget-Friendly

Breakfast:

- Oatmeal with Cinnamon and Sliced Bananas

Lunch:

- Rice and Black Bean Burrito with Salsa

Snack:

- Popcorn (seasoned with nutritional yeast)

Dinner:

- Baked Chicken Thighs with Roasted Vegetables

Tips for meal preparation and portion control

In order to support your metabolic health and maintain a healthy diet, portion control and meal preparation are essential.

Preparing Meals:

1. Arrange Your Meals: Make a weekly menu that consists of a range of well-balanced meals and snacks. Making healthier decisions and resisting the urge to order takeout can both be accomplished by planning ahead.

2. Cook in batches: Make more food and freeze it in portion-sized freezer bags. This simplifies the process of preparing nutritious, home-cooked meals in a pinch.

3. Incorporate a Variety of Foods: Try to incorporate a range of whole grains, fruits, vegetables, lean meats, and healthy fats into your meals. Variety guarantees that the nutrients you receive are varied.

4. Prepare Ingredients in Advance: To make meal preparation during the week easier, wash, chop, and prepare fruits, vegetables, and proteins in advance.

5. Use Healthy Cooking Methods: Steer clear of frying and instead use baking, grilling, steaming, or sautéing. These techniques are better for your metabolism and use less extra fat.

6. Limit Processed Foods: Reduce your intake of packaged and processed foods, which are frequently heavy in unhealthy fats, sodium, and added sugars.

7. Manage Portion Sizes: To prevent overindulging, serve meals in separate servings. Kitchen scales, portion control containers, and measuring cups are useful tools.

Control Point:

8. Visual clues: Estimate portion sizes based on visual clues. For instance, a cup of cooked pasta should be approximately the size of a tennis ball, a serving of meat should be around the size of a deck of cards, and a teaspoon of oil should be about the size of a poker chip.

9. Half-Plate Rule: Imagine cutting your plate in half and putting salad or veggies on one side and lean protein and whole grains on the other. Portion sizes are naturally regulated by this.

10. Incorporate Mindful Eating into Your Diet: Observe the signals your body sends when it is hungry or full. Consume food mindfully and gradually, since this can aid in avoiding overindulgence.

11. Use smaller plates and bowls: Using smaller plates and bowls when serving food can help manage portion sizes by giving the impression of greater quantities.

12. Pre-Portion Snacks: To prevent mindlessly consuming snacks from a bigger container, divide bulk snacks into single-serving portions.

13. Avoid Eating from the Container: Instead of eating straight out of packets, serve food on a plate or in a bowl. Portion size estimation is made simpler as a result.

14. Limit Liquid Calories: Pay attention to the number of calories in drinks. Instead of sugar-filled drinks, choose herbal tea, water, or other low-calorie options.

15. Check Food Labels: Examine food labels to determine serving sizes and the quantity of food included in a container. This will enable you to make wise decisions.

16. Restaurant Strategies: Share meals or get half servings when you're eating out. To limit your usage, request dressings and sauces on the side.

17. Track Your Intake:

Use a food diary or a smartphone app to track your daily food intake. You can identify patterns in your eating habits and maintain accountability by doing this.

18. Remain Consistent: Make an effort to continuously maintain portion control. Over time, this will become a habit that helps you manage your caloric intake and support your metabolic health.

CHAPTER FIVE

INCORPORATING PHYSICAL ACTIVITY

The role of exercise in boosting metabolism

Exercise is essential for increasing metabolism and enhancing general health. The processes through which your body uses the energy it receives from food to function are referred to as metabolism. Your metabolism can benefit from regular exercise in a number of ways:

1. Raise in Calorie Consumption: Calorie burning occurs during exercise, and the intensity of the exercise increases calorie burn. This contributes to the creation of a calorie deficit, which promotes fat reduction and weight management.

2. Maintaining and Building Muscle: Resistance training and strength training contribute to the preservation and growth of lean muscle mass. Having more muscle can raise your resting metabolic rate since muscle burns more calories when at rest than fat does.

3. The Effect of Afterburn (EPOC): Your body may undergo excess post-exercise oxygen consumption (EPOC) following a vigorous workout. This implies that as your body strives to replenish oxygen levels and repair muscle tissue, your metabolism stays high for a while after the workout.

4. Enhanced Sensitivity to Insulin: Frequent exercise will improve insulin sensitivity, which can facilitate your body's ability to control blood sugar levels. Those who are at risk of developing type 2 diabetes and insulin resistance may find this very helpful.

5. Increased Oxidation of Fat: Exercise can aid with weight management and body fat reduction by increasing the body's ability to use fat as an energy source.

6. Adaptations to Metabolism: Regular exercise can result in metabolic changes over time, including enhanced mitochondrial efficiency and function. The "powerhouses" of your cells, mitochondria, are in charge of generating energy.

7. Changes in Hormones: Exercise has an impact on hormones that are linked to metabolism. For example, it can cause the production of hormones like norepinephrine and adrenaline, which can momentarily increase metabolic rate.

8. Control of Appetite: Because exercise affects hunger hormones, it can help control appetite. It may also encourage healthier eating habits by raising your awareness of what you put in your mouth.

9. Heart Conditions: Enhancing cardiovascular health through exercise guarantees effective oxygen supply to bodily tissues and circulation. Metabolic processes may benefit from this.

10. Reduction of Stress: Stress can be effectively reduced by exercise. Elevated amounts of stress can trigger the release of cortisol, which may alter your body's energy storage and utilization. Exercise as a stress reliever can improve metabolic health.

11. Bone Health: Exercises involving weight bearing, such as strength training and walking, help preserve bone density, which is essential for general health, particularly as you age.

Safe and effective workouts for women over 50

For women over 50, safe and efficient exercise is crucial to preserving and enhancing general health, strength, and mobility. When creating an exercise program, it's critical to take your goals, your current level of fitness, and any underlying medical concerns into account. Here are some safe and efficient exercises designed specifically for women over 50:

1. Cardiovascular Exercise: Try to get 150 minutes a week of moderate-to-intense aerobic activity or 75 minutes a week of vigorous-to-intense aerobic activity. Dancing, swimming, cycling, and brisk walking are among the options. Increase intensity progressively after starting out softly.

2. Strength Training: Maintaining muscular mass, bone density, and metabolism requires strength training. Make use of bodyweight workouts, dumbbells, or resistance bands. Concentrate on your main muscular groups, including your back, legs, chest, and core.

3. Equations for Balance and Stability: Stability and equilibrium are more crucial as we get older. Include exercises that test your balance, such as heel-to-toe walking, standing on one leg, and yoga positions.

4. Stretching and Flexibility: Include consistent stretching activities to lower the chance of injury and increase flexibility. Every day, spend at least 10 to 15 minutes stretching your main muscle groups.

5. Yoga and Pilates: Pilates and yoga are great ways to strengthen your core, increase your flexibility, and balance. Additionally, these techniques aid in stress relief and relaxation.

6. Low-Impact Cardio: Low-impact exercises, such as swimming, water aerobics, or elliptical training, can offer a good cardiovascular workout with less strain on the joints if you have joint problems or are new to exercising.

7. Bodyweight Exercises: You can perform exercises like push-ups, planks, squats, and lunges at the gym or at home, depending on your level of fitness.

8. Circuit Training: Put together a circuit that combines aerobic, strength, and balance training. This makes your exercises engaging and difficult.

9. Interval Training: Include quick bursts of more intense activity in your aerobic routines. For instance, walk quickly for one minute and then more slowly for two minutes. This may enhance one's cardiovascular health.

10. Group Fitness Classes: Participating in group fitness programs, such as spinning, aerobics, or Zumba, can inspire people and foster a sense of belonging.

11. Functional Exercises: Concentrate on exercises that boost daily function, including step-ups to improve your ability to climb stairs or squats to improve sitting and standing.

12. Regular Warm-Up and Cool-Down: Always begin a workout routine with a warm-up to get your body ready for action, and end it with a cool-down to help your muscles relax and recuperate.

13. Speak with a Fitness Expert: Take into account collaborating with a personal trainer or fitness expert who specializes in working with senior citizens. They may offer direction, modify workouts to meet your needs, and guarantee correct form.

14. Listen to Your Body: Be mindful of any pain or discomfort you may be experiencing. If something about a workout doesn't seem right, adjust it or get advice from a fitness expert.

15. "Remain Hydrated and Get Enough Sleep: Recovery and general health depend on staying properly hydrated and getting enough sleep. Make sure you get enough sleep and consume enough water.

Creating an exercise routine that complements your diet

Developing an exercise regimen that works in tandem with your diet is a smart way to reach your fitness and health objectives. When properly paired, nutrition and exercise can enhance weight management, maximize metabolism, and enhance general wellbeing.

1. Set Your Objectives: Establish your fitness objectives, including weight loss, muscle gain, cardiovascular health, and general well-being. Your workout and food choices will be guided by your clearly defined objectives.

2. Take Your Diet into Consideration: Evaluate your present eating patterns and dietary requirements. Your fitness regimen should complement your nutritional objectives and meet your energy needs.

3. Balance Cardio and Strength Training: Include both strength training (such as bodyweight exercises and weightlifting) and cardiovascular activity (such as cycling, jogging, and walking). While strength training creates lean muscle, which can raise your metabolic rate, cardio helps burn calories.

4. Meal Timing and Exercise: Plan your workouts around your meals. Energy can be obtained by eating a well-balanced meal with protein and carbs one to two hours before working out. Have a post-workout meal or snack to help with muscle repair and recuperation after working out.

5. Hydration: Make sure you drink plenty of water prior to, during, and following physical activity. Hydration in moderation promotes overall performance and metabolism.

6. Incorporate Flexibility and Mobility Work: Frequent mobility exercises and stretches can increase your range of motion, lower your chance of injury, and improve the effectiveness of your workouts.

7. Variety and Progression: Use a range of exercises to keep your muscles from getting bored and to make sure all of your muscles are working. Increase the resistance, length, or intensity of your workouts gradually to push your body and encourage ongoing improvement.

8. Recovery and Rest: Allow your body enough time to recuperate in between sessions. Recovery is an essential part of any training program because it's when your body rebuilds and grows muscle.

9. Consult a Professional: To create a customized exercise program that complements your food and fitness objectives, think about speaking with a personal trainer or fitness expert.

10. Patience and Consistency: Seeing benefits from your workout regimen depends on consistency.

Recognize that reaching your objectives can take some time, and be patient while you make progress.

11. Record and Monitor: Maintain a fitness notebook to log your workouts and food consumption. This might assist you in determining what is effective and implementing the required changes.

12. Listen to Your Body: Observe how your nutrition and exercise affect your body. If you feel pain, discomfort, or extreme weariness, modify your routine and seek advice from a medical professional or fitness specialist as needed.

13. Periodic Assessment: Evaluate your food and exercise regimen on a regular basis to make sure they still meet your needs and growing goals. Make any necessary modifications.

CHAPTER SIX

MANAGING HORMONES FOR METABOLIC HEALTH

The influence of hormones on metabolism

Hormones play a crucial role in regulating metabolism, which encompasses all the chemical processes that occur within the body to maintain life. These hormones are produced and released by various endocrine glands and tissues and have a profound impact on how the body utilizes energy, stores fat, and manages blood sugar.

1. Insulin: Produced by the pancreas, insulin regulates blood sugar levels by allowing cells to take in glucose from the bloodstream and use it for energy. It also promotes the storage of excess glucose as glycogen in the liver and muscles. In this way, insulin influences both the utilization and storage of energy.

2. **Glucagon:** Also produced by the pancreas, glucagon has the opposite effect of insulin. It raises blood sugar levels by stimulating the release of stored glucose from the liver and increasing the breakdown of fats into usable energy.

3. Thyroid Hormones (T3 and T4): Produced by the thyroid gland, these hormones regulate the body's basal metabolic rate (BMR), which is the rate at which the body burns calories at rest. They control how cells use energy and affect processes like growth and development.

4. Cortisol: Released by the adrenal glands, cortisol is often referred to as the "stress hormone." It plays a role in glucose metabolism, inflammation regulation, and fat storage. Chronic stress and elevated cortisol levels can disrupt metabolic processes and lead to weight gain.

5. Leptin: Produced by fat cells, leptin helps regulate appetite and body weight. It sends signals to the brain about satiety and the body's energy stores, which influence food intake and metabolism.

6. Ghrelin: Secreted by the stomach, ghrelin is known as the "hunger hormone." It stimulates appetite and food intake, influencing energy balance and metabolism.

7. Adiponectin: Released by adipose (fat) tissue, adiponectin helps regulate insulin sensitivity, lipid metabolism, and inflammation. Higher levels of adiponectin are associated with improved metabolic health.

8. Epinephrine and Norepinephrine: These "fight-or-flight" hormones, produced by the adrenal glands, increase heart rate, blood pressure, and metabolic rate. They trigger the release of stored energy and enhance alertness and energy expenditure during stressful situations.

9. Growth Hormone (GH): Secreted by the pituitary gland, growth hormone influences growth and cell repair. It also affects metabolism by promoting the breakdown of fat for energy and the conservation of muscle tissue.

10. Estrogens and progesterone: These sex hormones, predominantly in females, influence fat distribution and insulin sensitivity. Changes in estrogen levels during menopause can affect metabolism and body composition.

11. Testosterone: Primarily a male hormone, testosterone also plays a role in regulating muscle mass, fat distribution, and overall metabolic health. Low testosterone levels in both men and women can impact metabolism.

Strategies to balance hormones naturally

Changing one's food and lifestyle to promote hormonal harmony is a natural way to balance hormones. The following techniques can assist in balancing and regulating hormones, though individual reactions may differ:

1. Modifications to Diet:

- **Ingredients:** Make eating a diet high in unprocessed, whole foods—like fruits, vegetables, whole grains, lean meats, and healthy fats—a priority. Limit or stay away from processed and sugary foods.

- **Fatty Acids Omega-3:** Include foods high in omega-3 fatty acids, such as walnuts, flaxseeds, and fatty fish (salmon, mackerel). Omega-3 fatty acids have anti-inflammatory and hormone-balancing properties.

- **Foods High in Fiber:** Eat a lot of fiber-rich foods, such as whole grains, legumes, fruits, and vegetables. Hormone and blood sugar balance are helped by fiber.

- **Healthy Fats:** Include foods high in healthy fats in your diet, such as almonds, avocados, and olive oil. These lipids are necessary for the synthesis of hormones.

- **Biological Estrogens:** Phytoestrogens found in some meals, such as flaxseeds and soy products, may help balance estrogen levels.

2. Regular Exercise: Take part in a regular physical activity regimen that combines cardiovascular, strength, and flexibility training. Exercise supports hormonal balance, lowers stress, and regulates insulin.

3. Stress Management: Engage in stress-relieving activities like yoga, tai chi, deep breathing exercises, or mindfulness meditation. Developing efficient stress management techniques is essential since long-term stress can upset hormone balances.

4. Adequate Sleep: Make sure you get between seven and nine hours of good sleep every night. Hormones that affect stress and hunger are among those that require sleep to be in balance.

5. Weight Management: Keep your weight in check with a well-balanced diet and frequent exercise. Hormonal abnormalities can result from excess body fat, particularly in the abdominal region.

6. Reduce Alcohol and Caffeine: Lessen alcohol and caffeine intake, as excessive amounts can disrupt the production and balance of hormones.

7. Hydration: Drink water all day long to stay well hydrated. Hormone transfer is one of the many body activities that are supported by adequate hydration.

8. Steer clear of endocrine disruptors: Reduce your exposure to environmental endocrine disruptors, like some of the chemicals in pesticides and plastics. When it's feasible, choose organic fruit and BPA-free containers.

9. Herbal Supplements: Certain herbal supplements, such as vitex (chasteberry), may assist with hormone regulation. See a medical professional before attempting any natural medicines.

10. Reduce Alcohol and Caffeine: Excessive intake of alcohol and caffeine might upset the balance of hormones. Restrict your consumption or go for healthier options like herbal tea and non-alcoholic drinks.

11. Meals that Support Hormones: Include meals that help with particular hormones. Broccoli and kale, for instance, are examples of cruciferous foods that can enhance estrogen metabolism.

12. Schedule Inspections: Seek routine medical examinations and think about hormone testing to find any imbalances. Talk to your healthcare professional about any worries you may have.

13. Lifestyle Changes: Take into account lifestyle choices like birth control or medication that can affect your hormones. If needed, go over alternatives with a healthcare professional.

The impact of menopause and hormone replacement therapy

The end of a woman's reproductive years is marked by the normal biological process of menopause. It is usually diagnosed between 45 and 55 years of age and is marked by a decrease in the production of progesterone and estrogen. The physical and general health of a woman can be significantly impacted by menopause. One way to control these effects is hormone replacement therapy (HRT), but it has advantages and disadvantages of its own.

The Menopause's Impact:

1. Night sweats and hot flashes: Hot flashes and night sweats are common in women and can be painful and interfere with sleep.

2. Membrane Alterations: During sexual activity, vaginal dryness, itching, and pain may result from the drop in estrogen levels.

3. Organ Function: Decreased estrogen levels during menopause can raise the risk of osteoporosis because estrogen maintains bone density.

4. Heart Conditions: Because estrogen helps to maintain healthy blood vessels, menopause is linked to an increased risk of heart disease.

5. Variations in Weight: Weight gain and changes in body composition might result from hormonal changes.

6. Cognitive and Emotional Shifts: Though they are not common, mood swings and cognitive abnormalities might happen to certain women.

7. Well-Being: A decrease in estrogen might affect one's libido and level of sexual satisfaction.

HRT (Hormone Replacement Therapy):

Hormone replacement therapy (HRT) involves menopausal women taking hormone-containing drugs (often progesterone and estrogen) to replace their diminishing hormone levels. HRT comes in two primary varieties:

1. Fertility Therapy (FT): Women who have undergone a hysterectomy—the removal of the uterus—are administered this.

2. Estrogen-Progestin Combination Therapy (EPT): In order to lower the risk of endometrial cancer, this is usually prescribed for women who have uteruses and contains both progestin and estrogen.

HRT Benefits:

- **Symptom Relief from Menopause:** Night sweats, vaginal pain, and hot flashes can all be effectively reduced or eliminated with HRT.
- **Better Bone Health:** HRT can help preserve bone mass and lower the chance of fractures and osteoporosis.

Heart Condition: According to certain research, hormone replacement therapy (HRT) may benefit heart health, especially if started soon after menopause.

HRT's Risks and Concerns:

Risk of Breast Cancer: Breast cancer risk may be modestly elevated by long-term EPT use.

Threats to the Heart: For certain women, HRT may raise their risk of stroke and blood clots.

Endometrial Cancer Risk: In women who have uteruses, the use of ET without progestin may raise the risk of endometrial cancer.

Digestive Disorder: Hormone replacement therapy may increase the risk of gallbladder disease.

Symptoms of Withdrawal: Menopause symptoms may reappear if HRT is stopped.

CHAPTER SEVEN

OVERCOMING CHALLENGES AND PLATEAUS

Dealing with common obstacles in metabolic health

Overall wellbeing depends on having a healthy metabolism, yet many people encounter frequent challenges that might make it difficult for them to maintain or enhance their metabolic health. These difficulties can differ from person to person; however, the following are some standard approaches to overcoming typical difficulties:

1. Sedentary Lifestyle:

Obstacle: A lack of physical activity can slow down metabolism and lead to weight gain.

Solution: To begin, make regular exercise a part of your schedule. Whether it's walking, cycling, dancing, or team sports, pick hobbies you enjoy. Aim for at least 150 minutes of moderate-intensity aerobic exercise per week as you gradually raise your level of activity.

2. Improper Dietary Decisions: Barrier: Poor eating practices, such as a diet heavy in processed foods, sugar-filled drinks, and excess calories, can have a detrimental effect on metabolic health.

Remedy: Switch to a well-balanced diet that prioritizes whole foods, such as fruits, vegetables, whole grains, lean meats, and healthy fats. Prioritize nutrient-dense foods, limit processed foods and added sugars, and exercise portion control.

3. Chronic Stress:

Difficulty: Extended stress might cause hormone abnormalities, disturbed sleep patterns, and binge eating.

Resolve stress by practicing mindfulness, meditation, regular exercise, and relaxation techniques. Make self-care a priority and schedule leisure and happy activities.

4. Lack of Sleep:

Challenge: Insufficient sleep can impact appetite hormones, resulting in weight gain and disturbances in metabolism.

Remedy: Try to get seven to nine hours of good sleep every night. Make sure your bedroom is cozy, stick to a regular sleep routine, and avoid engaging in stimulating activities right before bed.

5. Genetic Factors:

Obstacle: Some people may be more susceptible to metabolic problems due to their genetic makeup.

Solution: Although genetics cannot be changed, you can regulate your lifestyle to reduce the influence of hereditary variables. Prioritize a balanced diet and consistent exercise, and seek medical attention for any concerns you may have.

6. Medication Side Effects:

Difficulty: Certain drugs, like steroids or some antidepressants, can interfere with metabolism.

Remedy: If you think a drug is influencing your metabolic health, speak with your doctor. They can look at different therapies or ways to lessen the negative effects.

7. Hormonal Changes:

Obstacle: Menopause and thyroid problems are examples of hormonal abnormalities that might impact metabolism.

Remedy: See a medical professional for an accurate diagnosis and management of hormone-related problems. To manage these disorders, they can suggest medication or lifestyle alterations.

8. Inactivity at Work:

Barrier: Not getting enough exercise during the day can be caused by sedentary employment.

Solution: Look for methods to add movement to your daily schedule of work. Take brief breaks to walk, stretch, or perform easy activities. Think about changing the ergonomics of your workstation or getting a standing desk.

9. Lack of Accountability:

Barrier: A lot of people find it difficult to maintain accountability for their metabolic health objectives.

One potential solution could be to seek assistance from a healthcare professional, a licensed dietician, or a fitness trainer. You can stay on course with accountability from a supportive group or a professional.

10. Inadequate Education:

Challenge: It's possible that some people are unaware of the concepts of metabolic health and how to enhance it.

Remedy: Become knowledgeable about metabolic health by reading books, consulting credible sources, or speaking with medical experts. You can make wise decisions when you are well-informed.

Tips for breaking through weight loss plateaus

Although it might be discouraging, reaching a weight reduction plateau is a typical occurrence on the weight loss path. It could become more difficult to lose weight if your body adjusts to your early attempts. Take into account the following advice to overcome a weight reduction plateau:

1. **Reassess Your Calorie Consumption:** Your body may require fewer calories when you lose weight. Review your daily calorie intake and make any necessary adjustments in light of your goals, current weight, and level of activity.

2. **Monitor Your Nutrition:** To keep track of your daily caloric intake, use a food journal or a smartphone app. Make sure you're not eating too many calories without realizing it, especially from hidden sources like sugar-filled drinks or mindless nibbling.

3. **Diversify Your Diet:** Experiment with different foods and recipes to provide variation to your meals. Having a variety of foods can help avoid

boredom and lower the chance of overindulging due to meal monotony.

4. **Pay Attention to Nutrient Density**: Give top priority to foods high in vitamins, minerals, and fiber. These foods include important nutrients and can make you feel satisfied and full.

5. **Time and Frequency of Meals**: Try different meal times and quantities. Smaller, more frequent meals or intermittent fasting work well for some people. Discover a feeding schedule that suits your needs.

6. **Increase Your Protein Intake**: When losing weight, protein can keep you feeling full and help you preserve your muscle mass. Include foods high in lean protein, such as fish, chicken, tofu, or lentils, in your diet.

7. **Adjust Macronutrient Ratios**: Experiment with various macronutrient ratios to see if they help you restart your weight loss, such as by consuming more healthy fat or fewer carbohydrates.

8. **Include Strength Training**: Include strength training activities in your exercise regimen. Gaining muscle can help you overcome plateaus and boost your metabolism.

9. **Vary Your Exercise Routines:** Your body might have gotten used to the exercises if you have been performing them for a long time. To push your body, try new exercises or make your current routines more intense.

10. **Adequate Hydration:** Sometimes, dehydration is confused with hunger. Make sure you stay hydrated throughout the day to avoid mindless munching.

11. **Make Sleep a Priority:** Try to get 7-9 hours of good sleep every night. Hormones that control hunger and metabolism can be impacted by sleep deprivation.

12. **Reduce stress:** Prolonged stress might impede weight-loss attempts and cause weight gain. Use stress-reduction strategies such as yoga, deep breathing, or meditation.

13. **Avoid Late-Night Snacking:** To give your body enough time to fully digest food, try to finish eating at least a couple hours before going to bed.

14. **Speak with a Medical Professional:** If, after attempting a number of tactics, you are still unable to overcome the plateau, you might want to consult a qualified dietitian or other healthcare

professional for advice. They are able to rule out any underlying medical conditions and offer tailored advice.

15. **Remain consistent and patient:** Keep in mind that progress may not always be linear and that plateaus in weight loss are typical. Maintain your patience with the process and your commitment to your objectives.

Staying motivated and committed to your metabolic diet

It can be difficult to remain inspired and dedicated to your metabolic diet, but there are a few tactics that can support you in sustaining your motivation and accomplishing your fitness and health objectives:

- **Set Specific, Measurable, Achievable Goals:** Establish clear, attainable goals for your metabolic diet. Having well-defined goals will help you feel purposeful and directed.

- **Make a Plan:** Construct a well-organized food schedule that complements your metabolic diet. It is simpler to maintain your nutritional goals when you have a strategy in place.

- **Monitor Your Development:** Maintain a notebook in which you record your food consumption, exercise regimens, and any adjustments to your measurements or weight. Maintaining a progress log can serve as a source of motivation and accountability.

- **Celebrate Small Wins:** No matter how tiny your accomplishments may be, acknowledge and celebrate them. Every accomplishment, be it a successful workout or a healthy lunch selection, is a positive step.

- **Find an Accountability Partner:** Assist a friend or relative who also has similar dietary objectives. You can support one another, exchange stories, and ensure one another's accountability.

- **Remain Educated:** Continue to learn about exercise, diet, and metabolic health. You'll be more empowered and driven to make good decisions the more informed you are.

- **Visualize Your Success:** Picture how you'll look and feel after reaching your objectives for metabolic wellness. Visualization is a potent source of inspiration.

- **Ask for Professional Advice:** Speak with a medical professional or registered dietitian who specializes in metabolic health. They can provide you with encouragement and support, track your development, and provide you with tailored advice.

- **Set Rewards:** Create incentives for yourself when you accomplish certain goals with your metabolic diet. These incentives may serve as additional inspiration to stick with it.

- **Plan for Challenges:** Recognize possible roadblocks and devise plans of action to get beyond them. Even in the face of obstacles, you can stay on course with the support of this proactive strategy.

- **Mindful Eating:** In order to practice mindful eating, take time to enjoy every bite, pay attention to your body's signals of hunger and fullness, and refrain from overindulging emotionally.

- **Incorporate Variety:** Experiment with different foods and recipes to keep your diet fresh. Maintaining your diet and avoiding boredom can both be achieved with variety.

- **Social Support:** Participate in a community that is encouraging or join online communities that are devoted to metabolic health. It might be inspiring to connect with people and share your experiences.

- **Remain Consistent:** Long-term success depends on consistency. Follow through on your plan to develop a habit of regular exercise and a nutritious diet, even on days when you're not feeling very motivated.

- **Remember Your "Why":** Ask yourself why you initially began your metabolic diet. Remembering your "why" will help you stay motivated, whether it's to feel better, have more energy, or enhance your health.

- **Modify Your Plan as Required:** Be adaptable when it comes to your metabolic diet. Make changes to your plan to better suit your needs and tastes if you discover that some of its components aren't working.

- **Self-Compassion:** Treat yourself with kindness. Refrain from self-criticism and instead cultivate self-compassion when facing obstacles or disappointments.

CHAPTER EIGHT

LONG-TERM MAINTENANCE AND LIFESTYLE CHANGE

Sustaining a healthy metabolic diet as a long-term lifestyle

Making long-lasting adjustments to your eating habits is necessary to maintain a balanced metabolic diet as a way of life.

- **Put an emphasis on whole, nutrient-dense foods:** Eat a diet high in complete, unprocessed foods, such as whole grains, lean meats, fruits, vegetables, and healthy fats. These foods promote metabolic health and offer vital nutrients.

- **Equilibrium Macronutrient Consumption:** Aim for a macronutrient diet that is balanced, consuming proteins, fats, and carbohydrates in moderation. The precise ratios could change depending on your needs and objectives, but the foundation of metabolic health is a well-rounded diet.

- **Portion Control:** Watch how much you consume in order to prevent overindulging. Make use of smaller plates and get comfortable observing your body's signals of hunger and fullness.

- **Regular Meals and Snacks:** To maintain steady energy levels throughout the day, try to eat regular meals and include healthy snacks. This can lessen the chance of overindulging because of intense hunger.
- **Hydration:** To ensure that you are adequately hydrated during the day, drink a lot of water. The body's cues for thirst and hunger can occasionally be confused.
- **Planning and Preparing Meals:** To help you stay on track with your metabolic diet, prepare your meals and snacks ahead of time. When you're on the go, bring wholesome meals and snacks and prepare healthy options at home.
- **Mindful Eating:** Engage in mindful eating by appreciating every taste, being present while you eat, and being aware of your body's signals of hunger and fullness. When eating, stay away from devices and TVs.
- **Moderation, Not Deprivation:** Give yourself permission to treat yourself occasionally, but only in moderation. Steer clear of extremely restrictive

diets because they can be difficult to maintain over time.

- **Find Healthier Substitutes:** Look into healthier substitutes for the meals you love. For instance, pick whole-grain foods over processed carbs or fresh fruit in place of sugary snacks.

- **Remain Up to Date:** Keep learning about nutrition, metabolic health, and the most recent findings. Having knowledge can enable you to make sustainable and well-informed food decisions.

- **Support System:** Seek the assistance of friends and family who are as dedicated to a healthy metabolic diet as you are, or get involved in a supportive community. Motivating and encouraging words can come from discussing struggles and experiences.

- **Regular Physical Activity:** Keep up a regular exercise schedule that incorporates a variety of strength, flexibility, and cardiovascular exercises. A good metabolic diet is enhanced by regular physical activity.

- **Adaptability:** Be able to adjust to the ups and downs of life. If your schedule or circumstances change, you may need to modify your metabolic diet.

- **Set and Review Goals:** Consistently identify and assess your objectives related to metabolic health. This can support your long-term journey by keeping you motivated and focused.

- **Celebrating Achievements:** No matter how tiny, take pride in and acknowledge your accomplishments. Acknowledging your development can be a very effective motivation.

- **Regular Health Check-Ups:** Make an appointment for routine check-ups with a medical professional to keep an eye on your metabolic health and to quickly address any concerns or problems.

- **Self-Compassion:** Treat yourself with kindness. Instead of criticizing yourself when you face obstacles or disappointments, learn to be compassionate with yourself.

Strategies for maintaining a healthy weight and metabolism

It takes time and a combination of nutritional, lifestyle, and mental health techniques to maintain a healthy weight and metabolism.

1. **Balanced Diet:** Consume a range of whole foods as part of a balanced diet. Place a strong emphasis on entire grains, fruits, vegetables, lean meats, and healthy fats. Processed food, sugar-filled drinks, and high levels of bad fats should be avoided or consumed in moderation.

2. **Portion Control:** Be mindful of portion sizes to avoid consuming too much food. Take note of serving sizes and use smaller dishes, plates, and utensils.

3. **Regular Meals:** Consume meals and snacks on a regular basis to keep your energy levels steady. Later in the day, overeating may result from missing meals.

4. **Hydration:** Throughout the day, sip a lot of water. Maintaining hydration can aid in preventing overeating and boost metabolic activities.

5. **Mindful Eating:** During meals, cultivate mindful eating by appreciating each bite, being aware of your body's signals of hunger and fullness, and putting an end to outside distractions.

6. **Meal Planning:** Arrange your meals and snacks ahead of time to avoid impulsive purchases of less wholesome foods.

7. **Regular Exercise:** Take part in a regular physical activity program that incorporates flexibility, strength, and cardiovascular conditioning. Aim for 150 minutes or more a week of moderate-to-intense aerobic exercise.

8. **Consistency:** To increase your metabolism and gain lean muscle mass, stick to a regular exercise schedule.

9. **Adequate Sleep:** Try to get between seven and nine hours of good sleep every night. Hormones linked to metabolism and hunger can be affected by sleep deprivation.

10. **Stress Management**: To help manage stress and avoid emotional eating, try stress-reduction methods like deep breathing, meditation, or yoga.

11. **Regular Check-Ups:** Make an appointment for routine check-ups with a medical professional to assess your metabolic health, deal with any concerns, and get advice on keeping a healthy weight.

12. **Support System:** Assist yourself by interacting with friends, family, or a local organization. Having other people witness your journey can help you stay motivated and accountable.

13. **Set Achievable Goals:** Make attainable goals for your weight and health. Refrain from having unrealistic expectations, as this might cause irritation.

14. **Celebrate Achievements:** Honor all of your accomplishments, no matter how tiny. Acknowledging and rewarding yourself for your achievements can increase your drive.

15. **Education:** Keep learning about fitness, diet, and metabolic health on a regular basis. You can make wise decisions when you are well-informed.

16. **Self-Compassion:** Treat oneself with kindness, particularly in the face of difficulties or disappointments. Aim for self-improvement rather than self-criticism.

17. **Long-Term Perspective:** Recognize that it takes a lifetime to maintain a healthy weight and metabolism; there is no short remedy. Be tenacious and patient in your endeavors.

18. **Professional Guidance:** For individualized guidance and support, speak with a qualified nutritionist, personal trainer, or healthcare practitioner if you are experiencing challenges or have special needs.

Celebrating your successes and enjoying a vibrant life over 50

Enjoying a vibrant life after 50 and celebrating your accomplishments is a beautiful and well-deserved undertaking.

1. **Practice gratitude:** Consider your blessings at the beginning of each day. Having a positive outlook on life can make you enjoy it more.

2. **Maintain Active Living:** Take part in physical activities you enjoy, such as yoga, dancing, swimming, or walking, to stay physically active. Frequent exercise can raise vitality, elevate mood, and improve general wellbeing.

3. **Discover novel interests:** Take this opportunity to discover new passions, interests, and pastimes. Try your hand at cooking, painting, gardening, or any other enjoyable hobby.

4. **Vacation and Adventure:** Arrange vacations to places you've always wanted to see. It can be rewarding and enlightening to travel and experience different cultures.

5. **Cultivate Relationships:** Develop and fortify your bonds with loved ones and friends. With those you love, spend time together and make enduring memories.

6. **Seek Lifelong Learning:** Keep learning new things by reading books, taking online classes, or going to talks. The mind is kept engaged and active by learning.

7. **Practice self-care:** Set aside time for rest, meditation, or spa days as a priority for your own wellbeing. Taking care of oneself is crucial to general health.

8. **Healthy Eating:** Make sure your diet is nutrient-rich and well-balanced to support your health. Enjoy the process of making your meals and take pleasure in them.

9. **Celebrate Milestones:** Celebrate important occasions with delight and priceless memories, such as anniversaries or birthdays.

10. **Build a Good Self-Image:** Accept your age and value the knowledge and life experiences that come with it. The secret to living a happy life is self-acceptance and confidence.

11. **Embrace Nature:** Go outside and enjoy the beauty of nature, whether you're hiking, gardening, or just observing it.

12. **Community Involvement:** Join clubs and organizations that interest you, volunteer, or take part in local events to get more involved in your community.

13. **Remain Social:** Make new acquaintances and stay in touch with old ones to maintain an active social life. Being socially active is crucial for mental and emotional health.

14. **Plan for Retirement:** Make a retirement plan that will provide you with the financial stability and peace of mind you need to enjoy your golden years.

15. **Reflect and Set Goals:** Consider your life experiences and make fresh resolutions for the

future. Satisfaction and contentment can result from ongoing evolution and growth.

16. **Dress with Confidence:** Choose outfits that exude style, comfort, and confidence. Using your own style to express yourself can be liberating.

17. **Art and Creativity:** Use writing, music, or art to express your creative side. Expressing oneself creatively can be joyful and healing.

18. **Seek Professional Guidance:** Take into account speaking with medical professionals and experts who can assist you in managing and preserving your health and wellbeing as you get older.

19. **Maintain a Journal:** Write down your feelings, ideas, and experiences. This can be a fruitful method to consider your life's journey.

20. **Create New Adventures:** Push yourself to do new things and go on adventures, including visiting unusual places or picking up a new language.

CONCLUSION

To summarize, achieving a dynamic lifestyle beyond the age of 50 is not only possible but also quite gratifying. This stage of life offers a distinct chance for individual development, self-exploration, and the pursuit of longstanding aspirations and interests. By adopting an optimistic attitude, engaging in regular physical activity, and cultivating deep and meaningful relationships, individuals can fully enjoy the multitude of pleasures and opportunities that accompany the process of aging.

It is crucial to give priority to self-care, uphold a healthy lifestyle, and seek expert advice when necessary to promote ongoing well-being. Commending significant achievements and fostering connections with cherished individuals enhance the richness and significance of our existence. As we grow older, the knowledge acquired through years of experience becomes a valuable resource that may be imparted to others and effectively utilized in attaining fresh objectives and ambitions.

The secret to experiencing a dynamic life beyond the age of 50 rests in the capacity to adjust, accept change, and seize every opportunity. Every day presents a chance to relish the joys of life, discover uncharted territories, and forge enduring memories. By approaching the later stages of life with sincerity and a clear objective, one can experience profound satisfaction, serenity, and an appreciation for the abundance of experiences that life presents. Embrace this distinctive and exquisite stage of life, as it guarantees new opportunities and ongoing development, assuring that the future offers even greater things.